SCID-5-AMPD

STRUCTURED CLINICAL INTERVIEW FOR THE DSM-5® ALTERNATIVE MODEL FOR PERSONALITY DISORDERS

MODULE I

Structured Clinical Interview for the LEVEL OF PERSONALITY FUNCTIONING SCALE

Donna S. Bender, Ph.D. • Andrew E. Skodol, M.D.
Michael B. First, M.D. • John M. Oldham, M.D.

Interviewee/ID#: _____

Interview date: _____ _____ _____
month   day   year

Clinician: _____

SCID-5-AMPD

STRUCTURED CLINICAL INTERVIEW FOR THE DSM-5®
ALTERNATIVE MODEL FOR PERSONALITY DISORDERS

MODULE I

STRUCTURED CLINICAL INTERVIEW FOR THE
LEVEL OF PERSONALITY FUNCTIONING SCALE

Donna S. Bender, Ph.D.
Director, Counseling and Psychological Services, and
Clinical Professor of Psychiatry and Behavioral Sciences,
Tulane University, New Orleans, Louisiana

Andrew E. Skodol, M.D.
Research Professor of Psychiatry, University of Arizona College of Medicine,
Tucson, Arizona; and Adjunct Professor of Psychiatry, Columbia University College of
Physicians and Surgeons, New York, New York

Michael B. First, M.D.
Professor of Clinical Psychiatry, Columbia University College of Physicians and
Surgeons, and Research Psychiatrist, Division of Clinical Phenomenology,
New York State Psychiatric Institute, New York, New York

John M. Oldham, M.D.
Professor of Psychiatry,
Barbara and Corbin Robertson Jr. Endowed Chair for Personality Disorders,
Baylor College of Medicine, Houston, Texas

An overview of the Module I rationale, structure, and approach is presented in the
User's Guide for the SCID-5-AMPD. Please refer to that manual for proper procedure
for conducting the assessment.

Contents

GENERAL OVERVIEW FOR THE SCID-5-AMPD

I'm going to start by asking you some questions about yourself and about problems or difficulties you may have had. I'll be making some notes as we go along. Do you have any questions before we begin?

NOTE: Any current suicidal thoughts, plans, or actions should be thoroughly assessed by the clinician and action taken if necessary.

DEMOGRAPHIC DATA

How old are you?

GENDER: ___ Male ___ Female ___ Other (e.g., transgender)

Are you married?

> *IF YES:* **How long have you been married?**
>
> *IF NO:* **Do you have a partner?**
>
> > *IF YES:* **How long have you been together? Do you live with your partner? Have you ever been married?**
> >
> > *IF NO:* **Have you ever been married?**

IF EVER MARRIED: **How many times have you been married?**

Do you have any children?

   IF YES: **How many? (What are their ages?)**

With whom do you live? (How many children under the age of 18 live in your household?)

EDUCATION AND WORK HISTORY

How far did you go in school?

IF FAILED TO COMPLETE A PROGRAM IN WHICH INDIVIDUAL WAS ENROLLED:
Why did you leave?

What kind of work do you do? (Do you work outside of your home?)

Have you always done that kind of work?

   IF NO: **What other kind of work have you done in the past?**

What's the longest you've worked at one place?

(continued on next page)

EDUCATION AND WORK HISTORY (*continued*)

Are you currently employed (getting paid)?

> *IF NO:* **Why not?**

IF UNKNOWN: **Has there ever been a period of time when you were unable to work or go to school?**

> *IF YES:* **Why was that?**

Have you ever been arrested, involved in a lawsuit, or had other legal trouble?

CURRENT AND PAST PERIODS OF PSYCHOPATHOLOGY

Have you ever seen anybody for emotional or psychiatric problems?

> *IF YES*: **What was that for? (What treatment did you get? Any medications? When was that? When was the first time you ever saw someone for emotional or psychiatric problems?)**
>
> *IF NO:* **Was there ever a time when you, or someone else, thought you should see someone because of the way you were feeling or acting? (Tell me more.)**

Have you ever seen anybody for problems with alcohol or drugs?

> *IF YES*: **What was that for? (What treatment[s] did you get? Any medications? When was that?)**

Have you ever attended a self-help group, like Alcoholics Anonymous, Gamblers Anonymous, or Overeaters Anonymous?

> *IF YES:* **What was that for? When was that?**

Thinking back over your whole life, have there been times when things were not going well for you or when you were emotionally upset? (Tell me about that. When was that? What was that like? What was going on? How were you feeling?)

Begin Module I with the following questions to get a basic sense of the interviewee's view of self and the quality of interpersonal relationships.

PRELIMINARY QUESTIONS ABOUT VIEW OF SELF AND QUALITY OF INTERPERSONAL RELATIONSHIPS

The purpose of this interview is to explore different ways in which you see yourself, your basic approach to life, and how you interact with other people. Let's start with some general questions about how you are as a person:

1. **How would you describe yourself as a person?**

2. **How do you think other people describe you?**

3. **How do you generally feel about yourself?**

4. **How successful would you say you are at getting the things you want in life? (Like having a satisfying relationship, a fulfilling career, close friends?)**

(continued on next page)

5.   What are your relationships with other people like?

6.   Who are the most important people in your life? How do you get along with them?

7.   How well do you think you understand yourself?

8.   How well do you understand other people?

LEVEL OF PERSONALITY FUNCTIONING
Instructions

Personality functioning is distributed across a continuum. Central to functioning and adaptation are individuals' characteristic ways of thinking about and understanding themselves and their interactions with other people. An optimally functioning person has a complex, fully elaborated, and well-integrated psychological world that includes a mostly positive, volitional, and effective self-concept; a rich, broad, and appropriately regulated emotional life; and the capacity to behave as a well-related, productive member of a society.

The Level of Personality Functioning Scale (LPFS) is comprised of the following four domains:

Self Functioning

Identity (a component of self functioning): Experience of oneself as unique, with clear boundaries between self and others; stability of self-esteem and accuracy of self-appraisal; capacity for, and ability to regulate, a range of emotional experience

Self-direction (a component of self functioning): Pursuit of coherent and meaningful short-term and life goals; utilization of constructive and prosocial internal standards of behavior; ability to self-reflect productively

Interpersonal Functioning

Empathy (a component of interpersonal functioning): Comprehension and appreciation of others' experiences and motivations; tolerance of differing perspectives; understanding of the effects of own behavior on others

Intimacy (a component of interpersonal functioning): Depth and duration of positive connections with others; desire and capacity for closeness; mutuality of regard reflected in interpersonal behavior

Consider the complete Level of Personality Functioning Scale provided on the following pages and provide a global score between 0 and 4, using your clinical judgment based on information from the General Overview and the Preliminary Questions.

> **GLOBAL SCORE: _____**

Level of Personality Functioning Scale

Level of Impairment	SELF		INTERPERSONAL	
	Identity	Self-Direction	Empathy	Intimacy
0—Little or no impairment	Has ongoing awareness of a unique self; maintains role-appropriate boundaries.	Sets and aspires to reasonable goals based on a realistic assessment of personal capacities.	Is capable of accurately understanding others' experiences and motivations in most situations.	Maintains multiple satisfying and enduring relationships in personal and community life.
	Has consistent and self-regulated positive self-esteem, with accurate self-appraisal.	Utilizes appropriate standards of behavior, attaining fulfillment in multiple realms.	Comprehends and appreciates others' perspectives, even if disagreeing.	Desires and engages in a number of caring, close, and reciprocal relationships.
	Is capable of experiencing, tolerating, and regulating a full range of emotions.	Can reflect on, and make constructive meaning of, internal experience.	Is aware of the effect of own actions on others.	Strives for cooperation and mutual benefit and flexibly responds to a range of others' ideas, emotions, and behaviors.
1—Some impairment	Has relatively intact sense of self, with some decrease in clarity of boundaries when strong emotions and mental distress are experienced.	Is excessively goal-directed, somewhat goal-inhibited, or conflicted about goals.	Is somewhat compromised in ability to appreciate and understand others' experiences; may tend to see others as having unreasonable expectations or a wish for control.	Is able to establish enduring relationships in personal and community life, with some limitations on degree of depth and satisfaction.
	Self-esteem diminished at times, with overly critical or somewhat distorted self-appraisal.	May have an unrealistic or socially inappropriate set of personal standards, limiting some aspects of fulfillment.	Although capable of considering and understanding different perspectives, resists doing so.	Is capable of forming and desires to form intimate and reciprocal relationships, but may be inhibited in meaningful expression and sometimes constrained if intense emotions or conflicts arise.
	Strong emotions may be distressing, associated with a restriction in range of emotional experience.	Is able to reflect on internal experiences, but may overemphasize a single (e.g., intellectual, emotional) type of self-knowledge.	Has inconsistent awareness of effect of own behavior on others.	Cooperation may be inhibited by unrealistic standards; somewhat limited in ability to respect or respond to others' ideas, emotions, and behaviors.

Level of Personality Functioning Scale (*continued*)

Level of Impairment	SELF		INTERPERSONAL	
	Identity	Self-Direction	Empathy	Intimacy
2—Moderate impairment	Depends excessively on others for identity definition, with compromised boundary delineation. Has vulnerable self-esteem controlled by exaggerated concern about external evaluation, with a wish for approval. Has sense of incompleteness or inferiority, with compensatory inflated, or deflated, self-appraisal. Emotional regulation depends on positive external appraisal. Threats to self-esteem may engender strong emotions such as rage or shame.	Goals are more often a means of gaining external approval than self-generated, and thus may lack coherence and/or stability. Personal standards may be unreasonably high (e.g., a need to be special or please others) or low (e.g., not consonant with prevailing social values). Fulfillment is compromised by a sense of lack of authenticity. Has impaired capacity to reflect on internal experience.	Is hyperattuned to the experience of others, but only with respect to perceived relevance to self. Is excessively self-referential; significantly compromised ability to appreciate and understand others' experiences and to consider alternative perspectives. Is generally unaware of or unconcerned about effect of own behavior on others, or unrealistic appraisal of own effect.	Is capable of forming and desires to form relationships in personal and community life, but connections may be largely superficial. Intimate relationships are predominantly based on meeting self-regulatory and self-esteem needs, with an unrealistic expectation of being perfectly understood by others. Tends not to view relationships in reciprocal terms, and cooperates predominantly for personal gain.

Level of Personality Functioning Scale (*continued*)

Level of Impairment	SELF		INTERPERSONAL	
	Identity	Self-Direction	Empathy	Intimacy
3—Severe impairment	Has a weak sense of autonomy/agency; experience of a lack of identity, or emptiness. Boundary definition is poor or rigid: may show overidentification with others, overemphasis on independence from others, or vacillation between these. Fragile self-esteem is easily influenced by events, and self-image lacks coherence. Self-appraisal is un-nuanced: self-loathing, self-aggrandizing, or an illogical, unrealistic combination. Emotions may be rapidly shifting or a chronic, unwavering feeling of despair.	Has difficulty establishing and/or achieving personal goals. Internal standards for behavior are unclear or contradictory. Life is experienced as meaningless or dangerous. Has significantly compromised ability to reflect on and understand own mental processes.	Ability to consider and understand the thoughts, feelings, and behavior of other people is significantly limited; may discern very specific aspects of others' experience, particularly vulnerabilities and suffering. Is generally unable to consider alternative perspectives; highly threatened by differences of opinion or alternative viewpoints. Is confused about or unaware of impact of own actions on others; often bewildered about people's thoughts and actions, with destructive motivations frequently misattributed to others.	Has some desire to form relationships in community and personal life, but capacity for positive and enduring connections is significantly impaired. Relationships are based on a strong belief in the absolute need for the intimate other(s), and/or expectations of abandonment or abuse. Feelings about intimate involvement with others alternate between fear/rejection and desperate desire for connection. Little mutuality: others are conceptualized primarily in terms of how they affect the self (negatively or positively); cooperative efforts are often disrupted due to the perception of slights from others.

Level of Personality Functioning Scale (*continued*)

Level of Impairment	SELF			INTERPERSONAL	
	Identity	Self-Direction		Empathy	Intimacy
4—Extreme impairment	Experience of a unique self and sense of agency/autonomy are virtually absent, or are organized around perceived external persecution. Boundaries with others are confused or lacking.

Has weak or distorted self-image easily threatened by interactions with others; significant distortions and confusion around self-appraisal.

Emotions not congruent with context or internal experience. Hatred and aggression may be dominant affects, although they may be disavowed and attributed to others. | Has poor differentiation of thoughts from actions, so goal-setting ability is severely compromised, with unrealistic or incoherent goals.

Internal standards for behavior are virtually lacking. Genuine fulfillment is virtually inconceivable.

Is profoundly unable to constructively reflect on own experience. Personal motivations may be unrecognized and/or experienced as external to self. | | Has pronounced inability to consider and understand others' experience and motivation.

Attention to others' perspectives is virtually absent (attention is hypervigilant, focused on need fulfillment and harm avoidance).

Social interactions can be confusing and disorienting. | Desire for affiliation is limited because of profound disinterest or expectation of harm. Engagement with others is detached, disorganized, or consistently negative.

Relationships are conceptualized almost exclusively in terms of their ability to provide comfort or inflict pain and suffering.

Social/interpersonal behavior is not reciprocal; rather, it seeks fulfillment of basic needs or escape from pain. |

INTERVIEWER INSTRUCTIONS

Module I now continues with assessment of the four domains of personality functioning presented in the LPFS. Each of the four domains is comprised of three subdomains, each of which is rated on a five-point scale: **0 = "Little or no impairment," 1 = "Some impairment," 2 = "Moderate impairment," 3 = "Severe impairment," and 4 = "Extreme impairment."** Ask each subdomain screener question and as many questions for level determination as needed to determine the rating of functioning for that subdomain. The manifestations elicited from the interview questions should characterize the interviewee's general personality functioning. Some impairment in functioning may vary according to the individual's emotional state. For example, a person's ability to be empathic may decline significantly when the person is upset. The overall rating of functioning in that domain should thus reflect a clinical judgment about how often the person is emotionally upset.

For each question, ask for examples and elaboration until you have sufficient information to make a rating for that subdomain. If the interviewee is temporarily impaired (e.g., by Substance Intoxication, Substance Withdrawal, Delirium), administration of the interview should be postponed to a future time.

It is important to keep in mind that many individuals lack extensive, if any, insight regarding their personality functioning. Thus, negative answers to questions should not necessarily be construed as sufficient evidence for deciding that a level does not apply. For example, if the respondent replies "no" to "Do you think you are better, smarter, or more attractive than almost everyone else?" but consistently treats the interviewer in a very condescending and arrogant way, the latter behavior should be considered when posing additional questions and deciding on the appropriate level score. At the same time, higher levels of functioning may be endorsed by a lower-functioning interviewee without supporting evidence. For instance, someone might endorse being good at understanding others' perspectives but be unable to give supporting information or examples. All of the information gathered throughout this interview and the overall interaction with the individual should serve as data in determining the level of personality functioning.

Based on the response to the eight Preliminary Questions and the estimated global LPFS score, along with the interviewee's response to the screener questions, start the interview questions at the level where you think the interviewee may be functioning and continue from there for level determination.

Using the Sense of Self subdomain as an example, if it is fairly clear from the answers to the screener questions that the individual has at least moderate impairment (Level 2) in his or her sense of self, the interviewer should start with Level 2 probes. The interviewer should continue to ask questions corresponding to increasing levels of impairment until the interviewee clearly does not qualify for that level of impairment (i.e., it is clear from the assessment that a rating at a lower level of functioning is not applicable).

IDENTITY DOMAIN

Begin this section with:

You've told me some general things about how you see and feel about yourself, but I would like to ask you a bit more about that now.

Identity Domain **Sense of Self Subdomain**
Screener Questions: Do you sometimes have the experience of not really knowing who you are or how you are unique in the world? (Tell me about that.)   Do you sometimes find yourself wishing you were someone else? (Tell me about that.)

Circle subdomain rating	Level of functioning definition	Interview questions
0 = Little or no impairment	Has ongoing awareness of a unique self; maintains role-appropriate boundaries.	Do you almost always feel like you are your own person? Do you generally feel that where you are in your life makes sense to you?
1 = Some impairment	Has relatively intact sense of self, with some decrease in clarity of boundaries when strong emotions and mental distress are experienced.	Are you usually aware of who you are and what your perspective is? *IF YES:* **When you are upset, are you less aware? Give me some examples.**
2 = Moderate impairment	Depends excessively on others for identity definition, with compromised boundary delineation.	Do you depend on other people's opinions in order to know who you really are? Is it hard for you to know who you are without knowing what other people think of you?

Circle subdomain rating	Level of functioning definition	Interview questions
3 = Severe impairment	Has a weak sense of autonomy/ agency; experience of a lack of identity, or emptiness.	**Do you tend to feel empty much of the time?**
	Boundary definition is poor or rigid: may show overidentification with others.	**Do you sometimes completely lose the sense of who you are when interacting with others?**
		Do you often take on the emotions and ideas of people you identify with?
		When you are in an intense relationship with someone, do you often feel like you can't tell the difference between your feelings and the other person's or that you can't tell the difference between how you feel and how the other person feels?
	Overemphasis on independence from others, or vacillation between these.	**Do you sometimes have the feeling that you need to retreat from others to be your own person?**
		Do you find yourself needing to assert your independence in order to keep from feeling "swallowed up"?
4 = Extreme impairment	Experience of a unique self and sense of agency/autonomy are virtually absent, or are organized around perceived external persecution.	**Do you often feel that everyone around you is out to get you, take advantage of you, or persecute you?**
		Do you often need to protect yourself from being hurt or taken advantage of by other people?
	Boundaries with others are confused or lacking.	**Do you feel that most of the time you have no sense of who you really are?**

	Identity Domain	
	Self-Esteem Subdomain	

Screener Question:

What kinds of situations or people have the potential to affect how you feel about yourself? Tell me about that.

Circle subdomain rating	Level of functioning definition	Interview questions
0 = Little or no impairment	Has consistent and self-regulated positive self-esteem, with accurate self-appraisal.	**Would you say you feel pretty good about yourself most of the time?**
1 = Some impairment	Self-esteem diminished at times, with overly critical or somewhat distorted self-appraisal.	**Do you think you are excessively hard on yourself at times?** **Do you set goals or have expectations that end up making you feel like you don't measure up?**
2 = Moderate impairment	Has vulnerable self-esteem controlled by exaggerated concern about external evaluation, with a wish for approval.	**Does how you feel about yourself depend almost entirely on what others think of you?** **Do you feel bad about yourself if you don't get approval from others?**
	Has sense of incompleteness or inferiority, with compensatory inflated, or deflated, self-appraisal.	**Do you typically feel inferior to everyone else?** **Do you think you are better, smarter, or more attractive than almost everyone else?** **Do you think others often fail to understand your special qualities?**

Circle subdomain rating	Level of functioning definition	Interview questions
3 = Severe impairment	Fragile self-esteem is easily influenced by events, and self-image lacks coherence.	**Do you tend to feel bad about yourself very easily? Tell me about that.**
		When something doesn't go right for you, does it make you feel like you are a complete failure or loser?
	Self-appraisal is un-nuanced: self-loathing, self-aggrandizing, or an illogical, unrealistic combination.	**Do you at times feel that you are better than everyone else and at other times feel you are the worst? Do you sometimes have both of these feelings at the same time?**
		Do you often find yourself filled with shame and self-hatred?
		Have you had a lot of ups and downs or confusion in how you feel about yourself?
4 = Extreme impairment	Has weak or distorted self-image easily threatened by interactions with others; significant distortions and confusion around self-appraisal.	**Do you almost always feel bad about yourself no matter what is going on or what happens?**
		Do you almost always feel like bad things are happening to you? Tell me about that.

Identity Domain
Emotional Range and Regulation Subdomain

Screener Questions:

Are you an emotional person?

How do you deal with having strong feelings about things?

Circle subdomain rating	Level of functioning definition	Interview questions
0 = Little or no impairment	Is capable of experiencing, tolerating, and regulating a full range of emotions.	**Would you say you are comfortable with your feelings?** **Do you feel like you are able to experience the full range of feelings that people might have, like being excited, satisfied, really happy, angry, anxious, and sad?** **Are you okay feeling sad, annoyed, or angry at times?**
1 = Some impairment	Strong emotions may be distressing, associated with a restriction in range of emotional experience.	**Do you feel uncomfortable or upset if you get emotional about something?** **Do you try to keep your emotions "in check" because you don't like them to get out of hand?** **Do you think feelings just get in the way of being reasonable?**
2 = Moderate impairment	Emotional regulation depends on positive external appraisal. Threats to self-esteem may engender strong emotions such as rage or shame.	**Do you need others to appreciate or validate you in order to feel okay?** **Do you feel really bad, ashamed, or very angry if other people do not understand you or say bad things about you?**

Circle subdomain rating	Level of functioning definition	Interview questions
3 = Severe impairment	Emotions may be rapidly shifting;	Are you usually very moody and have a lot of ups and downs with your emotions?
	Or a chronic, unwavering feeling of despair.	Do you almost always feel really depressed, hopeless, or in despair?
4 = Extreme impairment	Emotions not congruent with context or internal experience.	Do you tend to have few or no feelings about situations that affect you, either good or bad?
	Hatred and aggression may be dominant affects, although they may be disavowed and attributed to others.	Do you usually feel angry, irritated, and hateful toward everyone around you?
		Does it seem like other people are always angry or hateful toward you?
		Can you describe situations in which that happens?

Identity Subdomain Scores

Record each <u>Identity subdomain</u> score here:

Sense of Self (pages 11–12)	_____
Self-Esteem (pages 13–14)	_____
Emotional Range and Regulation (pages 15–16)	_____
Sum these scores and divide by 3:	_____
	Record this average on page 36.

SELF-DIRECTION DOMAIN

Begin this section with:

Let's get back to the topic of how things are going for you in your life.

Self-Direction Domain
Ability to Pursue Meaningful Goals Subdomain
Screener Questions: Are you clear on what you want to accomplish for yourself in your life? Tell me about that.   Do you know how to get ahead?

Circle subdomain rating	Level of functioning definition	Interview questions
0 = Little or no impairment	Sets and aspires to reasonable goals based on a realistic assessment of personal capacities.	Do you have clear goals for the future? Do you generally feel like you have a good idea of what you need to do to move forward? Do you think you have what it takes to meet your goals in life?
1 = Some impairment	Is excessively goal-directed,	Is achieving your goals the most important thing to you? Do you typically devote most of your energy towards achieving your life goals rather than living in the present?
	Somewhat goal-inhibited,	Does needing to get things just right make it hard to set or achieve goals for yourself?
	Or conflicted about goals.	Is it hard to decide on your goals or which should be top priority?

Circle subdomain rating	Level of functioning definition	Interview questions
2 = Moderate impairment	Goals are more often a means of gaining external approval than self-generated, and thus may lack coherence and/or stability.	Is it important to you to achieve certain things so that other people will like you or approve of you? Have you pursued goals that other important people in your life disapprove of? Could you give some examples? Do you become confused about your goals if you aren't sure what others think you should do?
3 = Severe impairment	Has difficulty establishing and/or achieving personal goals.	Do you usually get really confused and overwhelmed when you think about trying to accomplish things in your life? Has it been hard for you to set or achieve goals in your life? Have you failed to do what needs to be done to achieve your goals?
4 = Extreme impairment	Has poor differentiation of thoughts from actions, so goal-setting ability is severely compromised, with unrealistic or incoherent goals.	Do you dream big dreams for your life but don't ever manage to take action? For example? Do you usually feel so overwhelmed that it is a challenge just to manage from day to day so that setting goals for the future is just too hard?

Self-Direction Domain
Constructive, Prosocial Internal Standards of Behavior Subdomain

Screener Questions:

Tell me about what kinds of standards you have set for yourself in terms of your behavior and morals.

Do you have a good idea about how you should behave and what you need to do to have a successful and fulfilling life?

Circle subdomain rating	Level of functioning definition	Interview questions
0 = Little or no impairment	Utilizes appropriate standards of behavior, attaining fulfillment in multiple realms.	**Does it feel like you have solid values and know what to do to get along with others and have a satisfying life?** **Do you think that you have a generally satisfying life?**
1 = Some impairment	May have an unrealistic or socially inappropriate set of personal standards, limiting some aspects of fulfillment.	**Are you typically perfectionistic or expect things of yourself other people might consider unreasonable?** **Do you have high personal standards that you need to stick to?** **Is it important to you to always follow your rules or values no matter how it might affect other people?**

Circle subdomain rating	Level of functioning definition	Interview questions
2 = Moderate impairment	Personal standards may be unreasonably high (e.g., a need to be special or please others) or low (e.g., not consonant with prevailing social values). Fulfillment is compromised by a sense of lack of authenticity.	Is it top priority for you to do things to please others or demonstrate that you are special? Is it important to you to create just the right impression to please others, or to get what you want? Are your values and ideals usually superior to most other people's? Do you think people should just get out of your way and let you do what you want? Are you willing to ignore the rules to get what you want?
3 = Severe impairment	Internal standards for behavior are unclear or contradictory.	Do you have a hard time trying to figure out whose values you should try to live by? Do you sometimes see clearly what your values are and how you want to behave, only to become quickly confused again? Do you feel like you are constantly failing yourself and others and there is no point in trying to do the right thing? Is life just too hard to know what is right or wrong?
	Life is experienced as meaningless or dangerous.	Do you generally feel that life is meaningless or dangerous?

Circle subdomain rating	Level of functioning definition	Interview questions
4 = Extreme impairment	Internal standards for behavior are virtually lacking. Genuine fulfillment is virtually inconceivable.	**Is life just an ongoing struggle to survive in any way you can?** **Are rules irrelevant in this dog-eat-dog world?** **Do you almost always feel like you have no idea about how you should act or what is expected of you?**

Self-Direction Domain
Self-Reflective Functioning Subdomain

Screener Questions:

How well do you know how your mind works—that is, how you think about things?

Is it hard to think about things when you become emotional or anxious?

IF YES: **Can you describe what that is like for you?**

Circle subdomain rating	Level of functioning definition	Interview questions
0 = Little or no impairment	Can reflect on, and make constructive meaning of, internal experience.	**Is it fairly easy for you to understand what is going on in your own head?** **Can you usually make constructive use of your thoughts and feelings?**
1 = Some impairment	Is able to reflect upon internal experiences, but may overemphasize a single (e.g., intellectual, emotional) type of self-knowledge.	**Do you tend to focus much more on how you think than on how you feel?** **How about the opposite…do you focus almost entirely on your feelings to the exclusion of everything else?**
2 = Moderate impairment	Has impaired capacity to reflect on internal experience.	**Is it often a challenge for you to figure out your mind, or what your perspective is on things?** **Do you need other people to give you input to be able to figure out what you are thinking and feeling?** **Do you often find that you don't know what you think or feel about something unless you bounce it off somebody else?**

Circle subdomain rating	Level of functioning definition	Interview questions
3 = Severe impairment	Has significantly compromised ability to reflect on and understand own mental processes.	Are you often pretty baffled about what makes you behave the way you do? Do you get confused when you try to figure out your own perspective or motivations? Do you often do things and act in certain ways without having any idea of why? Do your emotions take over you so you often can't even think straight?
4 = Extreme impairment	Is profoundly unable to constructively reflect on own experience. Personal motivations may be unrecognized and/or experienced as external to self.	Are you generally at a complete loss as to what you are thinking or feeling? Do you find that you are always on guard, reacting to what the world is throwing at you? Is it hard to think straight much of the time because everything is so uncertain and you have to worry about others harming or taking advantage of you?

Self-Direction Subdomain Scores

Record each Self-Direction subdomain score here:

Ability to Pursue Meaningful Goals (pages 17–18)	_____
Constructive, Prosocial Internal Standards of Behavior (pages 19–21)	_____
Self-Reflective Functioning (pages 22–23)	_____
Sum these scores and divide by 3:	_____
	Record this average on page 36.

EMPATHY DOMAIN

Begin this section with:

Let's talk some more about how well you think you understand other people.

Empathy Domain
Comprehension and Appreciation of
Others' Experiences and Motivations Subdomain

Screener Questions:

Is it easy for you to understand where other people are coming from?

How important is it to you to know what other people's concerns and experiences are?

Do you usually know what makes other people tick and why they do the things they do?

Have you found it easy to understand your partner in romantic relationships?

Circle subdomain rating	Level of functioning definition	Interview questions
0 = Little or no impairment	Is capable of accurately understanding others' experiences and motivations in most situations.	**Are you generally able to put yourself in other people's shoes?**
1 = Some impairment	Is somewhat compromised in ability to appreciate and understand others' experiences;	**Are you surprised that some people have such different opinions from yours?** **Do you often find it hard to appreciate how others feel about things and about you?**
	May tend to see others as having unreasonable expectations or a wish for control.	**Do you tend to feel that people expect too much from you?**

Circle subdomain rating	Level of functioning definition	Interview questions
2 = Moderate impairment	Is hyperattuned to the experience of others, but only with respect to perceived relevance to self.	Are you interested in what other people say or do mostly so you can take care of yourself and your own interests? Do you go out of your way to understand others so that you can stay in their good graces? What about going out of your way to know the proper thing to do? Do you need to know what is going on with them to make sure they are not thinking badly of you?
3 = Severe impairment	Ability to consider and understand the thoughts, feelings, and behavior of other people is significantly limited;	Is it hard for you to understand why people do things that hurt or upset you? Do you often find other people to be really confusing, unreliable, manipulative, or deceitful?
	May discern very specific aspects of others' experience, particularly vulnerabilities and suffering.	Are there certain people that you can see right through, that is, you immediately sense what is going on with them? Do you easily pick up on other people's pain?
4 = Extreme impairment	Has pronounced inability to consider and understand others' experience and motivation.	Do you find other people's motivations to be completely mystifying to you? Do most other people seem to do things without rhyme or reason? Is it just really hard to know what people will come at you with?

Empathy Domain
Tolerance of Differing Perspectives Subdomain

Screener Questions:

How do you deal with people who have opinions that are really different from yours?

How has it been for you if a partner or spouse has disagreed with you?

Circle subdomain rating	Level of functioning definition	Interview questions
0 = Little or no impairment	Comprehends and appreciates others' perspectives, even if disagreeing.	**Are you generally able to understand and appreciate other people's viewpoints when they disagree with you?**
1 = Some impairment	Although capable of considering and understanding different perspectives, resists doing so.	**Even if you can understand someone else's opinion, does it annoy you if they don't agree with you?** **Do you generally consider your way of doing things, or your perspective, to be the best or right way?**
2 = Moderate impairment	Is excessively self-referential; significantly compromised ability to appreciate and understand others' experiences and to consider alternative perspectives.	**Is it a top priority that your opinion is heard and appreciated by others?** **Is it boring to have to listen other people's stories and opinions?** **Do you generally find that other people's opinions are not worth listening to unless they agree with yours?** **Have you been told sometimes that you don't seem very interested in what other people have to say?**

Circle subdomain rating	Level of functioning definition	Interview questions
3 = Severe impairment	Is generally unable to consider alternative perspectives; highly threatened by differences of opinion or alternative viewpoints.	**Do you become really confused about your own ideas when someone else expresses a strong opinion?** **Is it upsetting or threatening to think that somebody you know could have really different ideas from yours?**
4 = Extreme impairment	Attention to others' perspectives is virtually absent (attention is hypervigilant, focused on need fulfillment and harm avoidance).	**Do you have to be very careful to protect yourself from other people because you never know where they might be coming from?** **Is it such a top priority to take care of yourself or guard against getting hurt that you never consider what other people think?**

Empathy Domain
Understanding of Effects of Own Behavior on Others Subdomain

Screener Questions:

How much impact do you think your actions have on other people?

Do you wonder sometimes why your partner or spouse reacts to you in certain ways?

Circle subdomain rating	Level of functioning definition	Interview questions
0 = Little or no impairment	Is aware of the effect of own actions on others.	**Are you usually aware of the effect of your actions on other people?** **If you hurt or offend someone, can you usually figure out what you did to cause that?**
1 = Some impairment	Has inconsistent awareness of effect of own behavior on others.	**Are you sometimes surprised or puzzled when people react in certain ways to things you do?**
2 = Moderate impairment	Is generally unaware of or unconcerned about effect of own behavior on others, or unrealistic appraisal of own effect.	**Are you generally not very concerned about how your actions affect other people?** **Are you surprised or upset when other people don't appreciate what you do?** **Is it most important to be able to do what you want when you want to do it regardless of the impact it has on others?** **Does it seem like almost everything you do impacts everyone else?** **On the other hand, do you think that no matter what you do, other people will be disappointed or disregard you?**

Circle subdomain rating	Level of functioning definition	Interview questions
3 = Severe impairment	Is confused about or unaware of impact of own actions on others; Often bewildered about people's thoughts and actions, with destructive motivations frequently misattributed to others.	Do you often find yourself in unpleasant or confusing situations with people? Can you give me some examples of this? Do people react to your behavior in ways that make no sense to you? Do people tend to get aggressive with you for no good reason? Can you give me some examples of this?
4 = Extreme impairment	Social interactions can be confusing and disorienting.	Are most people just better avoided so they don't hassle or take advantage of you in some way? Do you find that the ways people react to you leave you dumbfounded or disoriented?

Empathy Subdomain Scores

Record each Empathy subdomain score here:

Comprehension and Appreciation of Others' Experiences and Motivations (pages 24–25)	_____
Tolerance of Differing Perspectives (pages 26–27)	_____
Understanding of Effects of Own Behavior on Others (pages 28–29)	_____
Sum these scores and divide by 3:	_____
	Record this average on page 36.

INTIMACY DOMAIN

Begin this section with:

We have talked about some of your relationships. Let's get into that subject a little further.

Intimacy Domain
Depth and Duration of Connections Subdomain

Screener Questions:

Tell me about some important relationships you have in your life.
IF TALKS ABOUT ONLY FAMILY MEMBERS: **Do you have good friends outside your family?**

IF ONLY TALKS ABOUT ONE OR TWO PEOPLE: **Are there other people in your life you are close to?**

IF NO ROMANTIC RELATIONSHIPS HAVE BEEN MENTIONED UP TO THIS POINT: **Have you had satisfying romantic relationships?**

Circle subdomain rating	Level of functioning definition	Interview questions
0 = Little or no impairment	Maintains multiple satisfying and enduring relationships in personal and community life.	**Are there several people in your life that you have known a long time and feel close to?** **Do you feel like a valued member of your community?**
1 = Some impairment	Is able to establish enduring relationships in personal and community life, with some limitations on degree of depth and satisfaction.	**Do you feel like you have had a number of friendships in your life but sometimes they are not really that deep or satisfying?** **Are you too absorbed in your work, hobbies, or other activities to be able to spend enough time with friends or family?**
2 = Moderate impairment	Is capable of forming and desires to form relationships in personal and community life, but connections may be largely superficial.	**Do you feel like you have to put on a façade or that you are just playing a "role" in your relationships or your community life?** **Do you have a number of acquaintances, but feel like there is a lot missing in your connections?**

Circle subdomain rating	Level of functioning definition	Interview questions
3 = Severe impairment	Has some desire to form relationships in community and personal life, but capacity for positive and enduring connection is significantly impaired.	**Do you find you want to be in relationships, but a lot of times something happens to make them go wrong? Tell me about those relationships.** **Have you had a number of friendships or partnerships that have ended badly? Tell me about that.** **Have you had very few long-term friendships or relationships in your life?** **When you try to be a member of a group, do you often end up feeling on the outside or worried that people will see you as a bad or inferior person?**
4 = Extreme impairment	Desire for affiliation is limited because of profound disinterest or expectation of harm. Engagement with others is detached, disorganized, or consistently negative.	**Are you generally disinterested in relationships with other people?** **Do you usually feel detached or isolated from other people?** **Do you avoid relationships because you always end up getting hurt or taken advantage of?** **Are your relationships with other people generally negative?** **Do you mostly stay away from relationships altogether?**

Intimacy Domain
Desire and Capacity for Closeness Subdomain

Screener Questions:

Do you like to get to know other people?

Is it easy for you to open up in relationships?

Do you think you let other people get to know the real you?

Do you feel close to your spouse or partner? *(IF NOT CURRENTLY IN A RELATIONSHIP, ASK ABOUT RECENT PAST.)*

Do you and your partner know each other really well?

Circle subdomain rating	Level of functioning definition	Interview questions
0 = Little or no impairment	Desires and engages in a number of caring, close, and reciprocal relationships.	**Are you close to a number of people in your life?**
1 = Some impairment	Is capable of forming and desires to form intimate and reciprocal relationships, but may be inhibited in meaningful expression and sometimes constrained if intense emotions or conflicts arise.	**Is it a little difficult at times to be close with people if things get too emotional or disagreements arise?**
2 = Moderate impairment	Intimate relationships are predominantly based on meeting self-regulatory and self-esteem needs, with an unrealistic expectation of being perfectly understood by others.	**Is it important for you to try to get close to people so that you can feel appreciated or admired?** **Is it important to you to have friends or a partner whom other people admire?** **When you are in a friendship or relationship, do you get upset if that person doesn't understand you perfectly?**

Circle subdomain rating	Level of functioning definition	Interview questions
3 = Severe impairment	Relationships are based on a strong belief in the absolute need for the intimate other(s), and/or expectations of abandonment or abuse. Feelings about intimate involvement with others alternate between fear/rejection and desperate desire for connection.	**Do you feel lost if you are not in a close relationship?** **When you are in a relationship with someone you really care about, do your feelings alternate between needing a perfect connection and the fear that you are going to be rejected or abandoned?** **Do the people you form relationships with inevitably hurt or disappoint you?**
4 = Extreme impairment	Relationships are conceptualized almost exclusively in terms of their ability to provide comfort or inflict pain and suffering.	**Is it hard to trust people?** **Do you only interact with people when it's necessary to get what you need?** **Do you just mostly keep to yourself because others always end up hurting or taking advantage of you?**

Intimacy Domain
Mutuality of Regard Reflected in Interpersonal Behavior Subdomain

Screener Questions:

Do you find it easy to get along with most people?

Do you like to do things with friends and family?

Do you and your spouse or partner treat each other with support and respect? (IF INTERVIEWEE NOT IN A RELATIONSHIP RIGHT NOW, CAN ASK ABOUT RECENT PAST.)

Do you readily help each other out with chores, projects, and other responsibilities?

Circle subdomain rating	Level of functioning definition	Interview questions
0 = Little or no impairment	Strives for cooperation and mutual benefit and flexibly responds to a range of others' ideas, emotions, and behaviors.	Do you enjoy give-and-take in relationships and sharing experiences? Is it satisfying to work on projects and do activities with others?
1 = Some impairment	Cooperation may be inhibited by unrealistic standards; somewhat limited in ability to respect or respond to others' ideas, emotions, and behaviors.	Does it become hard for you to cooperate with other people when they don't share your standards? Do you tend to do things yourself so they get done correctly? Do you get impatient, frustrated, or bored if others' perspectives or reactions don't agree with yours?
2 = Moderate impairment	Tends not to view relationships in reciprocal terms, and cooperates predominantly for personal gain.	Do you primarily choose situations or relationships that clearly benefit you in some way, help you get ahead, or reflect well on you? Do you generally only do things with or for others if there is something in it for you?

Circle subdomain rating	Level of functioning definition	Interview questions
3 = Severe impairment	Little mutuality: others are conceptualized primarily in terms of how they affect the self (negatively or positively);	Do your relationships almost always end up one-sided so that most of the focus is on your needs rather than the other person's; or do you always end up taking care of someone else at your own expense?
	Cooperative efforts are often disrupted due to the perception of slights from others.	Is it hard to do things with others because it often feels like they disrespect you or don't meet your needs?
		Are your feelings easily hurt or do you feel too vulnerable when you are in group situations?
4 = Extreme impairment	Social/interpersonal behavior is not reciprocal; rather, it seeks fulfillment of basic needs or escape from pain.	Do you feel that most people just try to use you?
		Is it better just to avoid people altogether if they can't give you what you want or need?

Intimacy Subdomain Scores

Record each <u>Intimacy subdomain</u> score here:

Depth and Duration of Connections (pages 30–31)	_____
Desire and Capacity for Closeness (pages 32–33)	_____
Mutuality of Regard Reflected in Interpersonal Behavior (pages 34–35)	_____
Sum these scores and divide by 3:	_____
	Record this average on page 36.

MODULE I SCORING

All domains have now been assessed and scored. Next, determine the overall level of personality functioning score. Record the four domain scores according to their corresponding domain below. Total the scores, and then average the total to obtain the overall level of personality functioning.

Identity domain (page 16)	————
Self-Direction domain (page 23)	————
Empathy domain (page 29)	————
Intimacy domain (page 35)	————
TOTAL	_____
OVERALL LEVEL OF PERSONALITY FUNCTIONING (divide TOTAL by 4)	_____

EXPERTLY DESIGNED, the *Structured Clinical Interview for the DSM-5® Alternative Model for Personality Disorders* (SCID-5-AMPD) is a semi-structured diagnostic interview that guides clear assessment of the defining components of personality pathology as presented in the DSM-5 Alternative Model. The modular format of the SCID-5-AMPD allows the researcher or clinician to focus on those aspects of the Alternative Model of most interest.

Module I: Structured Clinical Interview for the Level of Personality Functioning Scale is devoted to the dimensional assessment of self and interpersonal functioning using the Level of Personality Functioning Scale. Module I provides both a global functioning score and an innovative, detailed assessment of all four domains of functioning (Identity, Self-Direction, Empathy, and Intimacy) and their corresponding subdomains.

Module I can be used independently or in combination with any of the following SCID-5-AMPD modules:

- **Module II** dimensionally assesses the five pathological personality trait domains and their corresponding 25 trait facets.

- **Module III** comprehensively assesses each of the six specific personality disorders of the Alternative Model, as well as Personality Disorder–Trait Specified.

Also available is the **User's Guide for the SCID-5-AMPD:** the essential tool for the effective use of each SCID-5-AMPD module. This companion guide provides instructions for each SCID-5-AMPD module and features completed samples of all modules in full, with corresponding sample patient cases and commentary.

Trained clinicians with a basic knowledge of the concepts of personality and personality psychopathology will benefit from the myriad applications and perspectives offered by the SCID-5-AMPD.

DONNA S. BENDER, PH.D., is Director, Counseling and Psychological Services, and Clinical Professor of Psychiatry and Behavioral Sciences at Tulane University in New Orleans, Louisiana.

ANDREW E. SKODOL, M.D., is Research Professor of Psychiatry at the University of Arizona College of Medicine in Tucson, Arizona, and Adjunct Professor of Psychiatry at Columbia University College of Physicians and Surgeons in New York, New York.

MICHAEL B. FIRST, M.D., is Professor of Clinical Psychiatry at Columbia University College of Physicians and Surgeons, and Research Psychiatrist in the Division of Clinical Phenomenology at the New York State Psychiatric Institute in New York, New York.

JOHN M. OLDHAM, M.D., is Professor of Psychiatry and Barbara and Corbin Robertson Jr. Endowed Chair for Personality Disorders at Baylor College of Medicine in Houston, Texas.

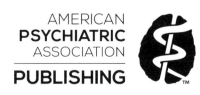

AMERICAN
PSYCHIATRIC
ASSOCIATION
PUBLISHING

WWW.APPI.ORG